Vitamin K2: Ultimate Guide About Vitamin For Living Healthy

Table of content

Introduction

It is important to understand what the structure of a vitamin is, then you can see how it serves the human body.

Vitamin K is a fat soluble vitamin and is primarily known for its blood clotting virtues, but with recent research indicating that vitamin K2 has further and more substantial benefits, such as helping to build strong bones and helping to prevent cardiovascular diseases, we also have to consider the importance of these new findings.

The human body is able to produce its own vitamin K2 from bacteria in the intestine as it turns vitamin K1 into vitamin K2. However, our body can only do this in small amounts and it may be insufficient to feel the full benefit of this vitamin. There are a number of ways you can increase this production, by the type of foods you eat, or even by taking supplements.

We will also go on to explain how beneficial vitamin K is to new born babies, so you can better understand why new borns are injected with vitamin K at birth.

It is also important to comprehend what conditions will clash with vitamin K and which medications might make your body low on vitamin K, such as:

Antibiotics.

Cholesterol medication.

Blood thinners, such as warfarin.

Now we have outlined the contents of this e-book, lets get started on learning in depth about the wonderful properties of vitamin K and exactly what the variants of this vitamin can do to make us live a healthy lifestyle.

Chapter 1 – What are Vitamins?

Let us first identify what exactly "vitamins"are and do, so we can go on to see why they are important to the human body.

Organisms

The human body is an organism, a life form. In order to be healthy, all life forms require certain essential nutrients to enable it to function correctly, and the human body is no different. The nutrients the human body needs to exist successfully, are broken down into a number of categories, such as

Carbohydrates

Fibre

Protein

Fat

Vitamins

It is the vitamins that this book is mostly concerned with, and especially Vitamin K2.

All these nutrients have something in common, chemical compounds. Those that have carbon, which is all vitamins, are also known as organic compounds. It is these compounds that help the body to successfully perform. Some life forms can create their own chemical, or organic compounds. These can vary as to what another life form can create for itself. For example, a dog can produce vitamin C but a human cannot, so for a human to benefit from vitamin C they would need to consume foods that contain it.

Vitamins are also made up of the separate elements called chemical compounds, but they are still organic substances, as they are natural atoms that gel together. These organic substances are present within other life forms, such as organic vegetation. They also contain a certain amount of carbon. All life needs carbon in some form, to survive. The human body needs carbon, but not in its purest form, so we obtain it through vitamins in our food.

Vitamins

Vitamins are just the same as the other nutrients in that they are made up of different atoms that gel together, with one of those atoms being carbon. It is the carbon in the nutrients that make them organic compounds. Carbon is an element which is present in all life forms.

Vitamins are generally classed into two different groups which are categorized on how they dissolve in your body.

<u>Fat-soluble Vitamins</u>

Fat soluble vitamins are stored in the fat tissues of the body. These are so named because they dissolve in fat. They are also stored in the liver once they have been absorbed through the digestive system. Because they are easy to store, they can be used as reserves and can be stored for days, and for some, even months. It also means that the stores can build up and become toxic, therefore when taken in excess they can be harmful for the host.

<u>Water-soluble Vitamins</u>

These types of vitamins are dissolved in water when they enter your system, and go directly to your blood stream. There is no way to store water soluble vitamins in your body. Because of this they do not stay in the body for long, and they are usually excreted via your urine. Hence, these need replacing regularly via your daily dietary intake. As water soluble vitamins are not stored in the body, they are generally non-toxic, no matter how much you ingest they will harm your body.

Common water soluble vitamins include –

Vitamin B1 (thiamine) Releases energy for the food we eat.

Vitamin B2 (riboflavin) Helps with healthy skin and good vision.

Vitamin B3 (niacin) Aids digestion.

Folic Acid helps promote healthy red blood cells.

C (absorbic acid) Protects cells and aids wound healing.

Fat soluble vitamins include -

Vitamin A is essential for healthy eyesight.

Vitamin D, increases the amount of calcium in the body and strengthens bones.

Vitamin E acts as an antidioxant in the body, which means it blocks other chemicals and starts a chain reaction, stopping unhealthy cells from going rampant.

Vitamin K (phylloquinone) is primarily known for its blood clotting abilities.

Chapter 2 – Vitamin K in Depth

Vitamin K was first identified in 1929 by a Danish Biochemist called Henrik Dam. While conducting experiments on chickens, investigating the functions of cholesterol, he isolated a compound that stopped the chickens from hemorrhaging, and called it *koagulationsvitamin*. This is now commonly known as vitamin K.

As previously mentioned, vitamin K is a fat-soluble type vitamin, and as it is not immediately used by the body, it is stored in the liver for future use. As with most vitamins, you only require a very small amounts every day, dependent on your body weight. The recommended dose is 0.001mg for every kilo of body weight. Therefore someone weighing 80 kilograms would need approximately 0.080 milligrams a day.

Vitamin K is an essential vitamin that helps the coagulation of our blood. It also helps to produce the necessary proteins that help to clot your blood, without vitamin k our blood be thin and would not clot. Those deficient in vitamin K show symptoms such as:

Excess and easy to bruise.

Profuse bleeding such as nose bleeds and bleeding gums.

Blood in faeces and in the urine.

Research is also highlighting that vitamin K has other benefits, such as helping with bone and kidney tissues. It helps to activate proteins that are needed to form new bone cells. Vitamin K helps to strengthen bones and reduce the risk of osteoarthritis, as shown in a study in 2013 which indicates that vitamin K deficiency is linked to knee osteoarthritis.

Types of Vitamin K

Vitamin K comes in three different forms:

Vitamin K1,

Phylloquinone, is the natural version and is found in plants and green leafy vegetables such spinach, kale and green leaf lettuce.

Phytonadione, is the synthetic type of vitamin K and is usually found in medication.

Phytonadione is available in the U.S. as vitamin supplement and can be purchased over the counter, without prescription, in 5mg tablets, or as a part of multivitamin tablets.

Vitamin K2,

Menaquinone, is the body's own vitamin K2, which is a product of the bacteria in your large intestine. Unfortunately most of this K2 produced is not available to the body, and therefore only provides a small amount of K2 for the body to use. Menaquinone is also obtained from foods such as meat, cheeses and eggs.

Vitamin K3,

Menaphthone, also known as meadione, is a synthetic based chemical and is a provitamin, meaning that it has no vitamin base, but the body converts it into a vitamin. In the case of K3, it is converted into K2.

Deficiency of Vitamin K

As previously suggested the recommended daily amount to digest is 0.001mg for each kilogram of body weight (65kg would require 0.065mg). It is rare for the human body to have a vitamin K deficiency, as bacteria in the human gut makes vitamin K. There are some health circumstances that can prevent the gut from absorbing vitamin K:

> Antibiotics can cause a temporary deficiency of this vitamin. The symptoms could be nose bleeds or bleeding gums.

> Blood thinning medication, such as warfarin. Those who are prescribed warfarin need to carefully balance their vitamin K intake, to ensure their levels do not fall too low. Neither can they have high levels as this will counteract the warfarin and thicken up the blood.

> Whilst vitamin K deficiency is uncommon in normal healthy adults, there are certain illnesses that can effect the levels of this vitamin in your body. Those with diseases such as, Liver, Gallbladder, Biliary, Cystic Fibrosis, Celiac and Crohn's, can be at risk from vitamin K deficiency.

> Serious skin burns can also effect the body's stores of vitamin K.

> A study has shown that long term Hemodialysis (kidney failure) patients have a reduced levels of Vitamin K.

Whilst there can be side effects from taking to much vitamin K, it is safe in the correct dosage and it is unlikely to cause harm to a healthy adult who takes up to 1mg a day.

Natural Forms of Vitamin K in Foods

There are many foods that are rich in vitamin K without the necessity of reverting to supplements. Most of us will get this vitamin through what we eat. The best types of food are the dark greens. A substance called Chlorophyll gives the vegetation its green color, and it is this substance that provides the vitamin K. It is important to include foods that are a natural source of vitamin k in your daily dietary intake, such as:

Kale

Dark green Cabbages

Spinach

Broccoli

Asparagus

Lettuce

Vitamin K can also be found in other foods, but to a lesser extent. These foods include :

Cauliflower

Fish

Eggs

Cheese

Cereals

Liver

Fruit

For the normal healthy adult it is not necessary to take supplements to ensure correct vitamin k levels. Simply eating a healthy diet with plenty of green vegetables, will provide you with all of the vitamin k your body needs to keep it healthy and fit.

Chapter 3 – The Functions of Vitamin K2

New evidence is indicating that the benefits of vitamin K2 go beyond just clotting the blood. Some scientists now believe that the vitamin K2 specifically, has many other benefits, such as:

Protects us from heart disease.

Keeps the skin healthy.

Makes bones stronger.

Promotes the function of the brain.

Prevents certain cancers.

Not only are scientists claiming that vitamin K2 has additional health benefits, but also, in many cases, vitamin K1 does not have the same effects.

A study, in the Netherlands, published in 2004, found that the best predictor of a patient more prone to heart disease was by the increased calcification of their arteries. The study found that those participants within the highest third of vitamin K2 intake not only had less calcification but were:

57 percent less likely to die from heart disease.

52 percent less likely to suffer from any calcification of their arteries.

41 percent less likely to ever develop heart disease.

Remarkably though, this study indicates that the benefits to reducing heart disease of those with high vitamin K2, were limited. In contrast, the intake levels of vitamin K1 showed none of the outcomes of increased protection from heart disease.

Benefits for Bones

There are frequent new studies now indicating the benefits of vitamin K2 on improving the health of our skeletal frame, with some early studies showing that vitamin K2 may also help osteoporosis. Studies are concluding that those with a high level of this vitamin have a greater bone density than those with lower levels, as is usually the case in those suffering from osteoporosis.

It can also help to strengthen the bones in post menopausal women, with a study showing that a daily intake of 45mg, combined with allium carbonate, showed and increase in bone density, compared to those who only took the calcium carbonate.

Further advantages that vitamin K2 imbues have been shown from studies regarding the calcification process. New claims are that vitamin K2 is used by different tissues, to deposit calcium and increase bone strength. This study shows that not only does vitamin K2 help direct the calcium to get to the right places, helping to strengthen bones and teeth, that it also stops calcium from depositing where it is not needed, more specifically in your arteries.

Cancer

As more studies are completed, scientists are becoming better convinced on the role of vitamin K2 as a means of added health benefits to bones, skin and prostrate health.

Increased intake of vitamin K2 is also now believed to reduce the risk of prostate cancer. Results of a study by the European Prospective Investigation into Cancer and Nutrition (EPIC) showed that there was a 35% lower risk of developing prostrate cancer, with an increase in vitamin K2. In this case and in comparison, the authors declared there was no reduction in risk with an increase in vitamin K1.

A Japanese study published in 2003 indicates that lung cancer patients given supplements of vitamin K2, along with other the anti-carcinogen drugs, such as Cisplatin, found the growth of lung cancer cells slowed down. These studies support previous work that has shown that vitamin K2 helps in treating Leukaemia.

The story of the benefits of vitamin K, in treating cancer, does not end here. This study in 2007 shows how patients with liver cancer, one of the deadliest forms of cancer, when given vitamin K with other anti-cancer agents, it suppressed the growth of liver cancer cells.

Diabetes.

Type 2 diabetes has often been called the modern western disease, as it is believed to be caused by a poor diet and a sedentary lifestyle, often associated with western lifestyle. It is a growing medical problem and one that impacts on the health care budget of many countries.

A study published in 2011 on healthy young men seems to indicate that an increase in the intake of vitamin K2, shows an improvement to insulin sensitivity, helping to reduce the risk of type 2 diabetes. Clearly one of the best ways to reduce your risk of diabetes type 2, is to be careful of what you eat and exercise regularly, but increasing your vitamin K2 intake may also help reduce the risk of contracting type 2 diabetes.

Scientists and food experts are agreeing that vitamin K2 should now be considered essential to the nutritional diet of humans. There are a number of natural food products that will help to boost your intake of Vitamin K2.

Foods with vitamin K2

There are a variety of foods from the culinary spectrum that are high in vitamin K2, and it is easy to eat a balanced nutritious diet, and one that will provide you with your daily amount of vitamin K2. Let us have a look at some of the sources:

One of the highest levels of vitamin K2 to be found is in a food known as Natto. This is a traditional Japanese fermented soybean and has approximately 0.775mg for every 100gm of Natto.

Dark chicken meat, such as thigh and drumsticks, there is more vitamin K2 in dark chicken meat than in chicken breast.

Most offal, kidneys, liver, brain and heart are high in vitamin K2.

Fermented vegetables, including sauerkraut, pickled cucumber, dill and Tempeh. It is the fermentation that increases the vitamin K2 in these products.

Fermented meat products, such as salami, calabrese and pepperoni, again it is the fermentation process that accounts for higher vitamin K2.

Certain cheeses, such as, Gouda, Jarlsburg, Edam and Brie, are high in vitamin K2. Other hard cheeses will also have vitamin K2, but not in the same quantities. Curd cheese and cream cheese is also a good source of vitamin K2.

Egg yolks and butter. An important element in the amount of vitamin K2 found in dairy produce and eggs, is if the source animal was grass fed. Eggs from free range chickens who feed on the pasture, will contain more vitamin K2 than those eggs that have been produced by factory farmed chickens.

Whilst it is possible for the human body to produce its own source of vitamin K2, which it does in the gastrointestinal tract, much of this K2 is not available for the body's use, and is therefore only a small amount. (Unden & Bonaerts, 19967, pp 217-234). Most of us get our vitamin K2 from the foods we eat, and that is why a diet rich in the foods mentioned above, is ideal for increasing your vitamin K2 intake.

Chapter 4 – Vitamin K for Newborn Babies

Babies

In the U.S. Canada, U.K. and other countries, new borns are automatically given an injection of vitamin K. In the US this practice has been in place since 1961. Whilst there can be some concern for the new parents, regarding injecting medicines into your new born baby, there is a very good reason for this.

New born babies are given vitamin K, because new borns have very small amounts of vitamin K in their system, and this is quickly used up. Because vitamin K is essential for blood clotting, it is given to new born babies to protect them from a rare, but serious disease called Vitamin K Deficiency Bleeding (VKDB). Approximately 1 in 10,000 new borns will be diagnosed each year with VKDB, meaning their blood will not clot. This leads to bruising and spontaneous bleeding from the nose or mouth, and other places. Sometimes this bleeding may not be visible, as it can also be internal in the brain and stomach. Children who have VKDB, clearly are seriously ill. Recently six infants were admitted to a the same hospital in the United States, after being diagnosed with VKDB. Four had serious bleeding to the brain, and two had internal bleeding to the stomach. The one thing they all had in common, was that none of their parents had taken the option to give the vitamin K injection at birth. Whilst fortunately, none of these children died, two of them required emergency brain surgery and one has serious brain damage, whilst two others have mild brain damage.

It is essential to have the vitamin K shot at birth, to protect your child from this dreadful disease.

VKBD can happen at any of the following three stages:

EARLY ONSET - within 24 hours after birth, this is very rare as most children are born with some vitamin K.

CLASSIC ONSET - within the first week of life, again this is rare

LATE ONSET - between 2-12 weeks after birth.

Whilst all these are rare, the LATE onset is even more unlikely, but it is the most serious. This onset is more likely to be the cause of internal bleeding, which cannot be seen and can lead to the brain hemorrhaging.

Babies who have had any sort of difficult birth are most at risk:

Born prematurely.
Needed assistance in birth, such as caesarean section or forceps.
Bruised in birth.
Breathing difficulties.
Liver problems.
Poorly at birth.
If the mother took drugs during pregnancy for epilepsy or tuberculosis.

Under normal circumstances breast fed milk is always encouraged, but in any of these situations, formula is better as it has a supplement of vitamin K. Even if the mother enriched her diet of vitamin K, this will only filter through in low amounts. Though breast milk gives so many other forms of extra protection. It is also known that feeding immediately after birth produces colostrum, which is rich in vitamin K, so this also helps.

For all of these reasons though, babies are automatically given vitamin K at birth. The risk is simply too great. Just one injection will see a baby through the risky first few weeks, while the natural immune system starts to build up.

Alternatively, vitamin K drops can be given orally, but any missed ones will leave baby at risk to the late-onset of VKDB. Giving drops is a little more complicated as it is calculated on whether baby is breast-fed or bottle-fed, and continues up to one month old.

At this point in the chapter, it is best to explain that there has been no evidence to prove that the vitamin K injection given to babies does any harm. Yet there is plenty of evidence to show all the benefits. It can be distressing for the parents seeing their newborn have the very first injection in life, but now you can understand a little better, why it is so necessary.

Chapter 6 – Recipes with Natto

Let us now have a look at the Japanese product called Natto. It is very nutritious and high in protein. Natto is basically, fermented boiled soybeans, and is a high source of vitamin K2. This process creates a bacterium known as Bacilus Natto. Natto is not present in any other soy foods, as this is a specific process. Natto has been used as a health food for hundreds of years by the Japanese. The Japanese intake of K2 is quite high and they have one of the highest levels of longevity than other nations, many see this as anything but a coincidence. It is not just longevity that the Japanese compare well to their western peers with, they have fewer blood clots, fewer deaths from cardio-vascular diseases and lower risk for certain cancers. In women, loss of bone density is at a slower rate than their western counterparts.

You can understand now why the Japanese believe that eating Natto has many health benefits, and helps to alleviate conditions such as:

VASCULAR -
Heart disease.
Blood pressure.
Stroke.
Hardening of the arteries as in deep thrombosis, such as varicose veins.

PAIN -
Endometriosis.
Fibroids.
Cancer.

Many argue that Natto is an acquired taste, some hate it and many love it. It has a powerfully pungent smell, not unlike that of a mature cheese. It has a strong taste and a slimy texture. In fact the smell for some is so overwhelming that some restaurants have separate Natto eating areas, to spare the other diners from its smell.

It is possible to make your own Natto, but it is a complicated process and does come in packets already made. For those who wish to try their hand at making it, the following recipe should work well.

Ingredients

2lb of Soybeans.
2 teaspoons of sterilized water.
1 spoon of Natto spores (it will have its own measuring spoon).
Large stainless steel pan and large stainless steel spoon.
Shallow glass containers, such as pyrex storage containers with plastic lids, 2 or 3 cup containers should be sufficient. If you haven't got containers with lids then large dishes covered with cling film should suffice.

It is essential that all equipment be thoroughly sterilized when it comes to the fermenting process. Any contaminants will stop the beans from fermenting.

Instructions

Wash the soybeans throughly and soak overnight in a water to bean ratio of 3 to 1, or 3 parts water to one part bean.

When soaked for at least 8 hours, drain the beans and add to the stainless steel pan. Cover with water and boil until soft. This should take around 6-7 hours.

Strain the beans and leave to stand, allowing them to cool slightly.

Add the Natto spores to two teaspoons of sterilized water, and stir with the sterilized spoon until mixed well.

Pour the Natto-spore infused water over the warm beans.

Mix thoroughly, ensuring the mixture is properly distributed amongst the beans.

Add the beans to your sterilized glass dishes, you don't want too many layers, around 2 inch depth of beans should be ideal. Cover the containers with lids or cling film.

Place the containers in a pre-heated oven of 100°f, for around 24 hours.

Remove the containers from the oven and stir thoroughly. Refrigerate for a couple of hours before eating. These beans will keep in the fridge for about a week and can be frozen if required.

Whether your Natto is store bought, or home made, let's get on and make some delicious recipes, using this nutritious ingredient.

NATTO RECIPES:

SOY NATTO

Ingredients

1 packet of Natto (ready done or home made)
1 tbspn of green spring onions (chopped)
1 tbspn of mustard of your choice
1 tbspn of dark soy sauce
3 Shiso leaves (can substitute with mint as hard to get hold of)

Method

Mix together the Natto, onions, mustard and soy sauce.

Serve on a bed of white steamed rice.

Garnish with the shiso leaves, or sprinkle with cinammon (which tastes similar).

NATTO BRUSCHETTAS

Natto's are ideal for topping the classic bread snack and can be combined in a number of ways.

<u>Cheese</u>

Serves 4

Ingredients

1 packet of Natto (ready done or home made)
1 French bread stick or other crusty bread
1 tablespoon of cream cheese
salt and pepper to taste

Method

Mix 5 tblspns of Natto with the cream cheese.

Season to taste.

Slice the bread into 8x 1/2 inch thick pieces.

Place the bread in a hot oven to crisp.

Once the bread is cool enough to handle, spread the Natto mixture on top.

<u>Tomato</u>

Serves 4

Ingredients

40g of Natto (ready done or home made)
1 French bread stick or other crusty bread
5 sweet cherry tomatoes
1/2 cup of onions (minced or grated)
2 tbspns of extra virgin olive oil
1/4 tspn of dry oregano

handful of fresh basil leaves
salt and pepper to taste

Method

Chop the Natto.

Chop the tomatoes.

Mix the Natto, tomatoes, onions, oregano, seasoning and oil.

Slice the bread into 8x 1/2 inch thick pieces.

Place the bread in a hot oven to crisp.

Once the bread is cool enough to handle, spread the Natto mixture on top and garnish with the fresh basil.

Chapter 6 – Possible Interactions with Vitamin K

There are certain medications that react badly to the presence of vitamin K:

ANTIBIOTICS

Patients on antibiotics have a reduction in the natural absorption of vitamin K. Antibiotics do not discriminate between good and bad bacteria, they kill bad bacteria, but also kill good bacteria that is needed to produce this vitamin. This is more so for patients taking antibiotics for more than 10 days, or taking cephalosporins, which include:

Cefamandole

Cefoperazone, also known as Cefobid

Cefmatazon, also known as Zefazone

Cefotetan

ANTICONVULSANTS

Patients who need medication for epilepsy, such as Phenytoin (also known as Dilatin), will find that this medication interferes with the absorption of vitamin K, so they will have a low dose of vitamin K.

BLOOD THINNERS

Because vitamin K blocks the effects of blood thinning medication, such as warfarin (also known as coumadin), these patients cannot take vitamin K supplements, and should also be careful eating foods known to have high levels of vitamin K (see chapter 3).

WEIGHT LOSS MEDICATION

Orlistat, also known as Xenical, is used for weight loss. It works by blocking certain chemicals in the gut, so they will not digest fat. This fat remains undigested and comes out in the stools, rather than being absorbed into your body. However, this medication also interferes with the absorption of vitamin K. Those patients using Orlistat or Xenical will need to take vitamin supplements.

There are certain foods that contain orlistat, and The Food and Drug Administration now require that such foods should have fat-soluble vitamins (K, A, D and E) added to these products.

CHOLESTEROL MEDICATION

Some drugs used to lower cholesterol levels, also reduce how much fat the body can absorb. This in turn will again reduce the absorption of fat-soluble vitamins, such as vitamin K, so a supplement may be required. These drugs are:

Cholestyramine, also known as Questran.

Colestipol, also known as Colestid.

Colsevelam, also known as Welchol.

Conclusion

I hope that now you have reached the end of this book you have a better understanding of vitamin K and in particular vitamin K2.

It is important to recognize nutrients and understand how they work within our own body's system. Once we know the best nutrients for ourselves, then we can make informed choice about what we eat, and in what quantities. Vitamin K2 is one such nutrient that can help our body stay healthy and strong

Now you know the benefits of an increase in vitamin K2, and the foods necessary to achieve this, hopefully you will be on the cusp of starting a new and healthy lifestyle. One that should help improve your bone density and reduce your risk of illnesses such as heart disease, cancer or even diabetes.

www.ingramcontent.com/pod-product-compliance
Lightning Source LLC
Chambersburg PA
CBHW070023260726
48658CB00003B/1017